Contents

What is the Pescatarian Diet?

A Pescatarian diet is a diet which excludes meat and poultry but includes plant foods, fish and seafood, dairy and eggs.

The word 'pescatarian' is a mix of the Italian word 'pesce' meaning fish, and the word vegetarianism. So, a Pescatarian diet includes lots of vegetarian recipes, but with the addition of fish. It is also very similar to the Mediterranean diet.

Other than the inclusion of seafood, there are no strict guidelines that determine what is pescatarian versus what is vegetarian. There are no rules that define how often you need to eat fish in order to be considered a pescatarian. For example, you may be a vegetarian who only occasionally eats fish or you may include it in every meal.

Pescatarians can get their protein from seafood, plant-based sources such as legumes, and sometimes, eggs and dairy products. This approach to eating can easily make for a balanced diet that provides all the necessary nutrients.

Choosing a pescatarian diet is a flexible way to modify a vegetarian diet. It adds the lean protein and omega-3 fatty acids offered by seafood to the health benefits of vegetables and fruit. A pescatarian diet is full of nutrient-dense, high-fiber, lower-calorie foods, so it could help those who have a goal of losing weight.

Aside from its health benefits, people opt for a pescatarian diet out of ethical concerns. From an ecological standpoint, pescetarianism lowers one's dietary carbon footprint. Livestock is the world's largest user of land, representing almost 80 per cent of agricultural land. The consumption of beef alone comprises 24 per cent of the world's meat intake.

The environmental impact and amount of energy required to feed livestock exceed its nutritional value. Unlike a vegetarian diet, pescetarianism provides a multitude of ways to keep your diet interesting.

Why a Pescatarian diet is better for the environment

"Reducing meat consumption has been shown to have a beneficial environmental impact," says Jenna. In fact, findings from an EAT Lancet study found foods that harm our health are also those that most harm the planet.

The most damaging food of all is red meat, like beef and lamb. For us, eating too much red meat can increase your risk of serious illnesses, like cancer, heart disease and stroke, and when it comes to our environment the figures are alarming. The study found, for example, that producing just 100g of beef results in 105kg of greenhouse gases – those emissions that are responsible for the greenhouse effect which has led to global warming. That's almost as many greenhouse gases as flying from London to Paris would produce.

"In order to optimise environmental impact it's recommended to switch animal-based foods for plant food sources," says Jenna. "The Pescatarian diet may be slightly more beneficial for animal welfare although it still encompasses dairy and animal-based products. Therefore, individuals with an ethical concern should generate their own views."

Foods You Can You Eat on the Pescatarian Diet

A balanced pescatarian diet includes fruits, vegetables, grains, legumes, and seafood. Most also include eggs and dairy products. A healthy pescatarian diet will often include flavorful foods such as olives, whole grains like farro and quinoa, spicy peppers, nuts, seeds, vegetable oils, and other nutritious, filling ingredients.

Unlike some other diets, a pescatarian diet is defined solely by compliant and non-compliant foods and ingredients. With no rules about portion sizes, components of meals/snacks, cooking methods, etc., an individual could follow a compliant diet that is very unbalanced. For instance, eating nothing Oreos, white rice, and beer-battered shrimp is not a healthy lifestyle despite that it is technically pescatarian. Keep this in mind as you design your meal plans, choosing real, whole foods over processed foods and limiting your intake of added sugars for a healthy, balanced diet.

What You Need to Know

The pescatarian diet is not a formal diet or weight loss plan, but rather a lifestyle. If you decide to be a pescatarian, you can eat meals and snacks whenever you prefer and as much as you prefer.

Of course, if you are looking to lose weight, portion control will be important. It's also a good idea to avoid overeating for long-term weight maintenance. When combined with regular exercise, a pescatarian diet that emphasizes nutrient-dense foods that are naturally lower in calories and fat could certainly help you lose weight and promote weight management.

If you have a health condition such as diabetes, celiac disease, or heart disease, a pescatarian diet is likely safe and probably beneficial. It's also pretty easy to avoid gluten on a pescatarian diet if you need to. But you should always check with your healthcare provider first and make sure that you're getting the right mix of nutrients for your body.

What to Eat

- Seafood

- Fruits and vegetables

- Grains

- Dairy products and eggs

What Not to Eat

- Red meat

- Poultry

- Wild game

Seafood

The seafood on a pescatarian diet may include freshwater fish such as trout or perch, saltwater fish like salmon or tuna, and shellfish including shrimp, oysters, clams, and more.

Dairy Products and Eggs

Most pescatarians eat eggs and dairy, although some do not. Technically, a pescatarian who eats eggs and dairy would be called a lacto-ovo-pescatarian.

Meat, Poultry, and Game

Regardless of whether or not you eat certain animal products like yogurt or cheese, if you follow a pescatarian diet you won't eat meat or meat products. That means you'll not only avoid red meat (like beef or bison) but you'll also avoid poultry, lamb, pork, and game (such as venison).

Sample Shopping List

A balanced pescatarian diet includes seafood, plant protein, fruits and vegetables, legumes, grains, or other complex carbs. As a great source of fiber, whole grains provide more nutrients and fewer sugars (and often, additives) than refined grains (like white rice and white flour).

There are no limits on the types of fruits and vegetables that can be included in this eating plan. Eat the rainbow and fill up on produce to receive the full health benefits; add dark leafy greens, bright red, yellow, and orange peppers, eggplant, corn, blueberries, kiwi, and other fruits and veggies.

If you buy fresh fish it usually needs to be cooked or frozen within a few days of purchase, so stock up on tuna packets or canned fish so you always have a seafood source ready to go. For more guidance, the following shopping list offers suggestions for getting started on the pescatarian diet. Note that this is not a definitive shopping list and you may find other foods and types of fish that work better for you.

- Dark leafy greens (spinach, kale, Swiss chard)

- Veggies (broccoli, cauliflower, Brussels sprouts, bell peppers, eggplant)

- Fresh and frozen fruits (grapefruit, oranges, berries, bananas, apples)

- Healthy fat sources (avocados, walnuts, almonds, chia seeds, olive oil)

- Whole-grains (100% whole wheat bread, brown rice pasta, quinoa, barley)

- Plant-based protein and legumes (tofu, soybeans, black beans, lentils, chickpeas)

- Canned or packaged fish (tuna, sardines, anchovies, salmon, herring)

- Fresh or frozen fish (halibut, cod, salmon, snapper, sea bass)

- Dairy products (cheeses, yogurt, milk, cottage cheese)

- Eggs

A Pescatarian Diet Meal Plan

For any of you starting on the pescatarian diet, it can be a discouraging task to prepare your meals. It's particularly easy to turn to lots of high carbohydrate meals, which isn't the best for anyone looking to maintain or enhance their wellbeing.

One of the benefits of the pescatarian diet is the heap of omega-3 fatty acids that you'll get from eating fish, which lowers inflammation. The pescatarian diet tends to have much lower levels of cholesterol which improves overall heart health.

So, if you're starting off this diet, give it a three-day trial.

Day 1

Breakfast

• Avocado Baked Eggs: a meal high in omega-3 fatty acids which means they're perfect as a breakfast meal, and they're packed with protein, fibre, vitamin C and A.

Lunch

• Moroccan Stuffed Sweet Potato Skins: a lunch meal that's filling. Sweet potatoes contain loads of Vitamin A and Vitamin C, so they're full of benefits. This recipe is packed with fibre and protein and low in fat.

Dinner

- Baked Tilapia with Parmesan Crust: is a pescatarians favourite. Baking the Parmesan as a crust really gives it a crunchy texture and the taste is mild enough that it doesn't overpower the flavour of the fish. Use a mix of olive oil and lemon juice to prep the fish before dipping it in the Parmesan mixture.

Day 2

Breakfast

- Huevos rancheros: a tasty Mexican breakfast meal loaded with carbs to get you through the day. If you want, you can serve the huevos rancheros up with some rice but a preferred method is to just have some flatbread or tortillas to eat it with.

Lunch

• Mackerel and green bean salad: make it with green beans, sugar snap peas and garden peas, so it's got a great crunch to it and has a zesty taste.

Dinner

• Teriyaki stir fry: a heavenly dish one can dine on. If you haven't got these exact ingredients in your refrigerator, no problem! Look for crunchy looking vegetables; carrots, cauliflower, bamboo shoots, bean sprouts and green beans and follow an online cooking recipe.

Day 3

Breakfast

- Avocado and sautéed mushroom toast: Avocado. Mushrooms. Sour Dough. Need I say any more? This is breakfast is right for anyone! If you'd rather tone down the carb intake then you can easily just remove the toast and it will still be delicious.

Lunch

- Greek chickpea salad: Chickpeas are a solid source of protein and they're one of those ingredients that boh stay fresh for a long time and are cheap to buy. I'd put them into the 'store cupboard essentials' category. They go perfectly with feta and tomato and that makes this salad simply delicious.

Dinner

- Red lentil curry and garlic and coriander naan: We eat a lot of lentils and this is curry, in particular, is one of our favourites. This is an optional side, but it's really tasty with lentil curry.

Enjoy it? Feel healthier? Then keep going! Here's a weekly diet pescatarian plan to follow:

Monday

- Breakfast: Any choice of cereal and a banana

- Lunch: Tuna salad

- Dinner: Tuna pesto pasta

- Dessert: 3x protein balls

Tuesday

- Breakfast: 2x blueberry & lemon muffins

- Lunch: Udon noodle soup

- Dinner: Sweet & sticky salmon kebabs

- Dessert: 4x carrot hummus cucumber cups

Wednesday

- Breakfast: Avocado baked eggs

- Lunch: Moroccan stuffed sweet potato skins

- Dinner: Thai massaman curry

- Dessert: Crème caramel

Thursday

- Breakfast: Coconut banana pancakes

- Lunch: Mac n cheese

- Dinner: Baked tilapia with a parmesan crust

- Dessert: Chocolate milkshake

Friday

- Breakfast: Weetbix & milk plus a banana

- Lunch: Mackerel & green bean salad

- Dinner: Teriyaki stir fry

- Dessert: Chocolate peanut butter protein ball

Saturday

- Breakfast: Avocado & sautéed mushroom toast

- Lunch: Greek chickpea salad

- Dinner: Beef or chicken burger

- Dessert: Ice scream

Sunday

- Breakfast: Fresh sardine fillets on toast

- Lunch: Veggie sub sandwich

- Dinner: Steak, mashed potatoes and veggies

- Dessert: Pudding

Pescatarian Snacks

If you're tight on time or just a not-that-bothered type, then you won't have to worry; pescatarian snacks don't require a ton of prep. Many of these alternative snacks are savoury and inexpensive. Here are some of the popular options you can enjoy at work or when you're at home:

- Sunflower seeds

- Roasted almonds

- Vegetable chips

- Museli bars

- Canned salmon

- Eggplant jerky

- Canned tuna

- Canned sardines

Can you lose weight on the Pescatarian diet?

Strictly speaking, the plant-based diet is not designed to help you lose weight. However, plant-based diets can aid weight loss. You may see drastic weight loss results if you follow a diet such as the 3-day Military diet, or the 5:2 diet, however these diet plans are not meant for the long term.

Rather, the Pescatarian diet promotes a sensible and healthy eating lifestyle. Though, you will be consuming far more vegetables than meat, and vegetables tend to have fewer calories and less fat. So, you'll be eating a diet naturally lower in calories and fat intake.

"Excluding meat and poultry will not necessarily lead to weight loss," says Jenna. "Weight loss comes down to what you are eating rather than what you're not. It is possible to obtain weight loss on a Pescatarian diet although simply adopting a Pescatarian diet will not lead to weight loss."

Other tips to lose weight while on the Pescatarian diet are avoiding frying your fish in oil, rather opt for healthier methods such as grilling or steaming your seafood.

Pros and Cons

Pros

• More protein choices than a strict vegetarian diet

• Health benefits

• Can be a good source of omega-3 fatty acids

• May have environmental benefits

Cons

• Can be expensive

• Watch for mercury levels

• May not always be caught or farmed sustainably

Some people who choose to eliminate meat from their diets may find that following a pescatarian diet is easier than following a strictly vegetarian diet because it is easier to get enough protein each day with the addition of seafood. When you replace meat-based meals with fish-based meals, you are likely to cut calories and fat from your diet to help you reach and maintain a healthy weight. Be sure to choose foods without added ingredients like sugar or salt whenever possible.

You'll also enjoy other wellness advantages if you choose this eating style. If you follow a pescatarian diet plan that is healthy and balanced, you get the benefits that are associated with a vegetarian diet, plus those associated with eating more fish.

The flexibility of this eating plan includes a wide array of compliant foods, with no specific limits on portion sizes and calories, which appeals to those who prefer a diet that is less regimented. However, the lack of specific guidance for making balanced, nutritious choices from compliant foods could pose a challenge to those who benefit from having a "rule book" to follow.

Additionally, buying the basic foods of this eating plan (fruits, vegetables, and fresh fish) can be costly. But you don't always have to buy fresh—many bulk bags of fruits and vegetables are just as healthy as the fresh versions. And frozen fish is easy to store and economical. Though canned tuna is minimally processed and contains sodium, it is perfectly healthy to consume in moderation.

Some people follow a pescatarian diet because of the positive impact certain seafood choices can have on the environment. Raising and processing meat takes up land and contributes to dangerous emissions. By reducing our dependency on meat and making sustainable fish choices, we do our part to help create a healthier planet.

Is the Pescatarian Diet a Healthy Choice for You?

Current guidelines set forth by the Department of Agriculture (USDA) suggest filling your plate with a balanced mix of protein (which could be from meat, fish, or plant-based sources), grains, fruits, vegetables, and dairy. The pescatarian diet meets that standard when meals are balanced with USDA-recommended foods and nutrients.

There's no official calorie count for the pescatarian diet, which means no need for calorie counting. However, the USDA suggests a daily calorie intake of about 1,500 calories for weight loss (although this number varies based on age, weight, sex, and activity level).

Regardless, the pescatarian diet features many low-calorie foods. If you're looking to lose weight, you may want to keep track of calories to create a healthy and sustainable calorie deficit. Use this calculator to determine the right calorie goal for you.

Health Benefits

Fish is low in saturated fat and rich in other nutrients. Fish is also a source of complete proteins, so you don't have to combine proteins to get the nutrients you need, but you will want to incorporate other healthy foods such as grains, vegetables, and legumes into your meals.

When you eat certain types of fish, you'll also boost your intake of omega-3 fatty acids. While some people take a supplement to get the recommended daily allowance, most health experts recommend that you get your intake from food. Omega-3 boosts heart health, may reduce symptoms of rheumatoid arthritis, and may even help to improve brain and eye health.

Studies have also shown that following a balanced vegan or vegetarian-based diet (including a pescatarian diet) is associated with lower body mass index (BMI). Other research suggests that people who follow a flexitarian diet (one that is primarily vegetarian but occasionally includes meat or fish) enjoy benefits including healthy body weight, improved markers of metabolic health, blood pressure, and reduced risk of type 2 diabetes.

Health Risks

Vitamin B12 is an important micronutrient typically found in animal foods, which means you may get less of it when you eat a pescatarian diet. B12 (cobalamin) helps to maintain a healthy nervous system, and aid in the formation of red blood cells and DNA and protein metabolism. Make sure you get plenty of meat-free foods high in B12 such as shellfish, eggs, milk, and dairy products, and some fortified cereals.

You'll also want to avoid fish with higher levels of mercury, especially if you are pregnant or breastfeeding. The Food and Drug Administration (FDA) and the Environmental Protection Agency (EPA) categorize fish into "best choices," "good choices," and "fish to avoid." Their resources are aimed at helping consumers make healthy and safe decisions when choosing seafood so they can reduce their intake of harmful toxins.

PESCATARIAN DIET RECIPES

Trying new pescatarian-friendly recipes is a great way to explore new flavors and find new favorite dishes while looking after your health. In this part are nourishing pescatarian diet recipes for you to enjoy.

Creamed cod

Preparation time

40 minutes

Ingredients

- 1kg of well-soaked stockfish (whole cod, beheaded and air dried by cold winds)

- 300g of extra-virgin olive oil

- 5 cloves of garlic

- Salt

Instructions

- Up to a day before you make the dish, slice the garlic cloves and place them in a bowl with the olive oil to give it an aromatic depth of flavour.

- Cut the stockfish into two or three pieces and steam it in a steamer for 15 mins.

- Once it has cooled down, remove skin and bones, and chop it well.

- Put the chopped stockfish in a bain-marie (a bowl over half a pan of hot water) and beat long and vigorously with a wooden spoon, gradually adding a little aromatic oil until creamy.

• Alternatively, use a blender.

• The fish essentially has to absorb all the oil until it's fluffy. If need be, add half a ladle of cooking water. Season to taste.

To serve

1. Serve the creamed cod on polenta croutons, with boiled sliced potatoes, on toasted bread or corn tortillas.

Herring under a fur coat

Preparation time

40 minutes

Ingredients

- Carrots 500g

- Beetroot 500g

- Potatoes 500g

- Mayonnaise 200g

- Onions 200g

- Salted herring fillet 500g

- 2 hard-boiled eggs

- Greens for decoration

- Salt and ground black pepper to taste

Instructions

1. Wash, peel and boil the potatoes, beets and carrots until tender.

2. Remove the skin and bones from the fish fillets and cut into small cubes. Or just use the fillets as they are.

3. Moisten the bottom of a bowl or plate and lay out the herring in an even layer.

4. Chop the peeled onion finely, scald it with boiling water, squeeze out the moisture and spread it over the fish.

5. Generously cover with mayonnaise.

6. Cut the boiled potatoes into small squares and put them in the next layer. Add a thin layer of mayonnaise.

7. Grate the carrots and beets separately on a coarse grater. Add the carrots and then the beetroots, heavily coated with mayonnaise.

8. You can repeat the layers, if you like.

9. Top the salad with chopped egg yolks or decorate with beetroot or carrot roses, sprigs of herbs, etc.

Serving

1. Cover the bowl with cling film and place in the fridge for several hours. At the table, cut the salad like a cake or jellied meat, into roughly equal pieces, or just spoon it onto plates.

Tuna melt with ketchup

Preparation time

25 minutes

Ingredients

• Tuna melt

• One 6-ounce (160 g) tin of tuna (preferred pole & line caught and MSC certified) in sunflower oil, drained

• 1 small red onion, diced

- 1 spring onion, white and light green parts, finely chopped

- ¼ bunch of flat-leaf parsley, leaves only, coarsely chopped

- 3 tablespoons mayonnaise

- Tabasco sauce

- 4 slices of bread, preferably rustic

- 1½ tablespoon (20 g) butter

- 4 slices of cheddar cheese

- Salt and pepper, to taste

Ketchup

- 2 tablespoons olive oil

- 1 garlic clove, minced

- 1 small red onion, diced

- One 14-ounce (400 g) can peeled plum tomatoes

- 1½ tablespoon tomato purée

- 1 tablespoon dark brown sugar

- 1 tablespoon red wine vinegar

- Salt and pepper, to taste

Instructions

1. Mix the tuna, onion, scallion, parsley, mayonnaise, and a few drops of tabasco in a bowl. Season with salt and pepper. Set aside.

2. To prepare the ketchup: Heat the olive oil in a saucepan over medium-high heat and sauté the

garlic and onion until soft but not browned, about 2 to 3 minutes, stirring frequently. Add the peeled tomatoes, tomato purée, sugar, and vinegar. Cook over low heat until thickened, about 3 to 5 minutes. Season the ketchup with salt and pepper. Press the sauce through a fine sieve and leave to cool.

3. Butter each slice of bread on one side and turn over. Pile the tuna mixture onto the non-buttered sides of two slices of bread and top with the cheddar. Cover with the other two slices (buttered side up).

4. Bake the toasted sandwiches for 2 to 3 minutes on each side in a dry frying pan over medium heat until the bread is crunchy and the cheese has melted.

5. Cut the tuna melt diagonally and serve with the ketchup.

Lobster diavola

Preparation time

35 minutes

Ingredients

- 1 tin of MSC Lobster meat

- 300g of fresh pappardelle, or spaghetti

- Cup of cherry tomatoes

- 1 cup of tomato passata

- 1 sprig of rosemary

- 1 tsp of chilli flakes

- Garlic cloves, finely chopped

- As much parmesan as you'd like

Instructions

1. Preheat your oven to 350F/180C degrees.

2. Toss your cherry tomatoes in olive oil and fresh rosemary, and bake them for about 15 mins until they're soft and tender.

3. Bring a large pot of salted water to a boil.

4. Heat a little olive oil in a large frying pan.

5. When hot, add in your garlic and sweat it off until it's tender.

6. Add in the tomato passata to your frying pan and let it reduce for approximately 5 minutes.

7. Add your pasta to the water, and let it cook until just tender. Reserve 1 cup of water.

8. Toss roasted cherry tomatoes in your frying pan, and add in your pasta.

9. Let everything cook together until the noodles are coated.

10. Check the sauce's consistency.

11. Add in a bit of your pasta water, if you'd like a thinner sauce.

12. Open one tin of Scout's butter poached lobster and add to the pan.

13. Stir gently to distribute the lobster and warm through.

14. Garnish with a few chilli flakes, fresh rosemary, and grated parmesan.

Shrimp cocktail al pastor

Preparation time

1 hour 15 minutes

Ingredients

For the cocktail sauce

- 4 tbsp homemade mayonnaise

- 1 tbsp mezcal

- 2 tbsp ketchup

- 2 tbsp cream a

- few drops of chipotle sauce

For the pineapple al pastor

- 1/2 pineapple

- 3 cloves of garlic

- 1 tbsp oregano

- 1 tbsp ground cumin seeds and black pepper

- 2 cloves

- 3 red chilies

- 50 ml white wine vinegar

- 50 ml pineapple juice

- 1 tbsp grape seed oil

For the pico de gallo

- 1 tomato

- few leaves chopped coriander

- ½ sweet onion

- ½ red chilli without seeds

- 1/4 pineapple

- juice of 1 lime

For the crispy filo

- 5 sheets of phyllo/filo dough

- 3 tbsp clarified butter

- A few leaves of lettuce

- 2 eggs

- 200g MSC certified shrimps/prawns

Instructions

1. Half beat the cream.

2. Mix the mayonnaise with the mezcal, ketchup and chipotle sauce. Fold the whipped cream into the cocktail sauce.

3. Keep in the fridge.

4. Preheat the oven to 180° C.

5. Heat the oil in a pan, add the garlic and fry until golden brown. Then add the oregano, cumin, cloves and black pepper.

6. Bake for 30 seconds. Set aside.

7. Fry the red chilies in the same pan.

8. Add the pineapple juice and vinegar and reduce to a slightly thicker mass. Add the garlic mixture to this.

9. Mix until smooth.

10. Cut the pineapple into wedges and mix into the mixed pasta so that every piece is covered with it.

11. Cook in the oven until the pineapple chunks are golden brown caramelized.

12. For the pico de gallo, cut all the vegetables and the pineapple into brunoise.

13. Mix with the juice of the lime and the coriander.

14. Season with salt and pepper.

15. Rub the sheets of phyllo dough with clarified butter.

16. Arrange all the sheets on top of each other and cut out circles with a serving ring that have the same diameter as the glass in which you serve the cocktail (or slightly smaller).

17. Bake the filo circles between two baking trays until nicely browned, about 10 minutes.

18. Boil the eggs for 5 minutes.

19. Cool in cold water.

20. Compose the cocktail: arrange a few leaves of lettuce in each glass.

21. Spoon some pico de gallo and cocktail sauce on top. On top of that, place half an egg and sprinkle with shrimp.

22. Arrange the cubes of pineapple 'al pastor' on top and cover the glass with the crispy filo pastry.

Tuna and olive stuffed romano peppers

Preparation time

45 minutes

Ingredients

- 1 small red onion, diced

- 1 small garlic clove, minced

- 12 shiitake mushrooms, chopped

- Half a 2-ounce (45 g) tin of sustainable anchovies, drained

- One 5-ounce (140 g) tin of tuna (preferred pole & line caught and MSC certified) in olive oil, drained

- 2 teaspoons capers

- 5 black olives, halved

- 2 romano peppers, halved

- 2 teaspoons panko (Japanese bread crumbs)

- Zest of 1 lemon

- ¼ bunch of flat-leaf parsley, leaves only, finely chopped

- Olive oil

- Pepper

Instructions

1. Preheat the oven to 350°F (180°C).

2. Heat a splash of olive oil over medium-high heat and saute the red onion, garlic, and shiitake mushrooms until softened, 3 to 4 minutes.

3. Add the anchovy fillets and let them "melt" in 2 minutes.

4. Finally, mix in the tuna, capers, and olives and cook for a few more minutes until warmed through.

5. Meanwhile, brush the halved peppers with olive oil and place them in an ovenproof dish.

6. Remove the tuna mixture from the heat, fill the peppers with it, and dust with panko.

7. Drizzle some extra olive oil on top and bake in the oven for 20 to 25 minutes, until crisp and done.

8. Scatter the lemon zest and the parsley over the peppers.

9. Season with freshly ground black pepper and serve.

Sweet curried lobster salad

Preparation time

25 minutes

Ingredients

Lobster salad

- 700g MSC certified lobster tails

- Half of an red onion, diced

- 1 celery stalk, finely chopped

- 10 cherry tomatoes, quartered

- Half of a green pepper, diced

- 1-2 green chillies, chopped

- 1 avocado, diced

- Shredded lettuce

Dressing

- 2-3 tbsp. mild curry powder

- 3 tbsp. brown sugar

- 2-3 tbsp. boiling water

- 5 tbsp. Mayonnaise

- Juice of half a lemon

- Salt and pepper to taste

Instructions

1. Bring a large pot of water to a boil.

2. Once the water is boiling, add 3 tablespoons coarse sea salt, then add lobster tails.

3. Cook for 8 to 10 minutes only, then remove from pot and set aside to cool down.

4. Once the tails have cooled down, cut them open down the centre of the tail and remove the meat.

5. Gently breaking the piece of meat in half will expose the vein which can now be easily removed.

6. Chop roughly and add to the rest of the salad ingredients.

7. For the dressing, add the curry powder and brown sugar to a mixing bowl.

8. Add the boiling water (just enough to dissolve), then add Mayonnaise, lemon juice, salt & black pepper and combine well.

9. Combine all salad ingredients except the avocado and lettuce.

10. Add the lobster and dressing and give it a good stir to get everything coated, then add the avocado.

11. Line a fancy glass with the shredded lettuce and place the salad onto the lettuce.

12. Serve and enjoy!

Fish finger fish

Preparation time

30 minutes

Ingredients

- 1 bread roll (e.g. a submarine roll)

- 3 MSC certified fish fingers

- 3 tbsp peas (fresh or frozen)

- 1 tbsp cream cheese

- 1 tbsp vegetable oil

Instructions

1. Heat the oil in a pan.

2. Fry the frozen fish fingers for 8 minutes, turning them over regularly.

3. Bring a small bowl of water to the boil and then add the peas.

4. Cook the peas for 5 minutes or until they are cooked.

5. Drain the peas and leave them to cool.

6. Mix the peas and cream cheese with a hand blender.

7. Cut off the two round ends or edges of the bread roll.

8. Using a small sharp knife, cut a mouth into one of the ends and create a tail shape with the other.

9. Create two sandwiches by cutting each end in half and cover the top half with pea/cream cheese blend.

10. Carefully push a skewer through the fish fingers and the sandwiches to create a fish shape.

Wild prawn larb

Preparation time

30 minutes

Ingredients

- 8 x MSC certified cooked king prawns (look for the blue fish tick), peeled and deveined, chopped roughly

- 300g green papaya, shredded

- 2 fresh mangoes, flesh only in rough chunks

- 150g snake beans or green beans, cut into 2cm lengths

- 1 Lebanese cucumber, sliced lengthways

- 1 cup of coriander

- 1 cup of mint leaves

- 1 cup of Thai basil leaves

- 2 kaffir lime, thinly sliced

- 1 baby gem lettuce, leaves picked for cups

- Pork floss, to serve (optional)

Fragrant prawn powder:

- 150g glutinous rice

- 4-5 thin slices galangal

- 4 kaffir lime leaves, coarsely torn

- 1 lemongrass stalk, thinly sliced

- Reserved prawn shells

Dressing:

- 80ml lime juice

- 60ml fish sauce

- 1 long fresh red chilli, seeded and finely chopped

- 3tsp ginger, finely grated

- 4tbsp palm sugar, crushed or softened in the microwave

Instructions

1. To make the prawn powder, preheat the oven to 175C.

2. Place all the ingredients onto a tray and roast for 15 mins or until the rice is golden.

3. Allow to cool before grinding in a spice grinder or mortar and pestle.

4. For the dressing, mix all of the ingredients into a bowl.

5. Place the prawn rice powder, chopped prawns, green papaya, mango, snake beans, cucumber and herbs in the dressing and toss to coat.

6. To assemble, place the lettuce cups onto the serving platter, pile up the prawn salad on top and pour extra dressing.

Serving suggestion

1. Garnish with kaffir lime and pork floss and serve immediately.

Shrimp salad sandwiches

Preparation time

15 minutes

Ingredients

- 50 g shrimps

- 6 slices of toasted bread

- 1/2 tbsp mayonnaise

- 3 halved sun-dried tomatoes

- 1 tsp parsley, finely chopped

- salt and pepper

Instructions

1. Mix the shrimps, mayonnaise, sun-dried tomatoes and parsley in a bowl.

2. Season with salt and pepper.

3. Cut out six fish shapes from the slices of toasted bread.

4. If you have one, you can instead use a fish-shaped cookie cutter.

5. Place a black sesame seed as the eye on each fish shape.

6. Use the fish shaped toasted bread to make shrimp salad sandwiches.

Wild Prawn Salad with Citrus and Avocado Emulsion

Preparation time

36 minutes

Ingredients

- 500 g MSC certified sustainable prawns (look for the blue fish tick)

- 1 tablespoon olive oil

- 1 tablespoon butter

- 250 g mayonnaise (see below)

- 4 avocados

- 60 ml lime juice

- 2 corn cobs

- 5 large tomatoes, pulp removed and diced

- 1/2 iceberg lettuce, finely shredded

- 1/4 cup fresh coriander leaves

- micro herbs (optional)

- sea salt

- black pepper

- 2 limes, halved

For the coriander mayonnaise

- 200 ml olive oil

- 200 ml avocado oil

- 2 teaspoons Dijon mustard

- 4 free range egg yolks

- 45 ml lime juice

- 1/4 cup fresh coriander leaves

- sea salt

- black pepper

Instructions

1. Heat some salted water in a small saucepan.

2. Cut corn cobs in half and add to water.

3. Reduce heat to a simmer and cook for 10-12 minutes.

4. Remove from the water, drain and set aside.

5. De-seed the tomatoes and chop - set aside.

6. Thinly shred the iceberg lettuce - set aside.

7. Remove the corn kernels from the cobs - set aside.

8. Using a blender, combine the avocados, lime juice and seasoning in a jug. Blitz until smooth.

9. Set aside in the fridge, in a bowl covered with cling wrap touching the top of the avocado.

10. Combine all the ingredients for the mayonnaise apart from the oils in a jug or blender.

11. Blitz for 10 seconds before slowly adding the oils while continuing to blend.

12. Once all the oil has been added or when it becomes a mayo consistency you like, remove from the jug or blender and set aside.

13. Remove the shells of the prawns.

14. Add the oil and butter to a large saucepan on medium/high heat.

15. Add the prawns and cook for 2-3 minutes on each side or until cooked through.

16. Remove from the pan and allow to cool down.

17. Once cooled, chop the prawns and combine with mayonnaise.

18. Assemble the stacks in eight parfait glasses with the avocado emulsion on the bottom, followed by the diced tomatoes, corn kernels, and lettuce.

19. Top with the prawns in mayo and micro herbs.

Salmon, cream cheese and cucumber bites

Preparation time

20 minutes

Ingredients

- 1 slice of smoked salmon (MSC or ASC certified)

- 1 slice of brown bread

- 1 tsp cream cheese

- 10 stems of chives

- Black peppercorns

- Radishes and cucumbers (for decoration)

Instructions

1. Toast a slice of bread.

2. Once toasted cut the shape of a fish body out of the bread.

3. Spread cream cheese on the fish body.

4. Cut the smoked salmon into 4 strips and cut off a wider piece for the tail.

5. Place the salmon strips onto the fish body and place the wider piece at the tail end.

6. Place the stalks of chives very close to the salmon strips.

7. Place a peppercorn as the fish eye.

8. Decorate with radishes and cucumbers.

Hake and potato stew

Preparation time

45 minutes

Ingredients

- 500g MSC certified hake fillets, cut into portions

- Olive oil

- Coarse ground sea salt and black pepper

- 1 teaspoon paprika

- 1-2 large onions, finely chopped

- 3-4 cloves of garlic, finely chopped

- 1 sprig of fresh rosemary, finely chopped

- 150ml white wine

- 8-10 baby potatoes, left whole

- 10-15 cherry tomatoes

- 250ml cream

- 400ml fish or vegetable stock

- 1 lemon, juiced

- 3-4 sprigs of fresh parsley, finely chopped

Instructions

1. Place the hake portions into a dish and drizzle with olive oil.

2. Season the fish with the salt, pepper and paprika, making sure each portion is evenly coated. Set aside.

3. Heat a little olive oil in a heavy bottomed casserole and brown the hake by searing it skin-side down.

4. Remove the fish from the pot and set aside.

5. If necessary, pour a little more olive oil into the pot and fry the onions until soft and translucent.

6. Add in the garlic and rosemary and fry for the further minute.

7. Deglaze the pot with white wine and add in the potatoes and tomatoes.

8. Sauté for a minute or two then pour in the cream and stock.

9. Stir the pot to combine and leave the stew to simmer for 15-20 minutes or until the potatoes and tomatoes are soft and cooked through.

10. Add the hake portions and the lemon juice and leave the potjie to simmer for a further 5 minutes.

11. Gently stir through the chopped parsley and serve the potjie with lots of crusty bread and white wine.

Steamed hake with sea lavender and gnudi

Preparation time

30 minutes

Ingredients

- 480g MSC certified hake fillet (approx. 120g per person)

- 500g ricotta

- 50g parmesan

- 2 lemons

- Flour

- 4 eggs

- Semolina

- Butter

- 4 handfuls of sea lavender

- 20 sage leaves

- Pepper

- Salt

Instructions

1. Grate the parmesan and mix with the ricotta along with the zest of 1 lemon. Use a peeler to remove the skin of the other lemon.

2. Save these for later.

3. Roll balls of the ricotta mixture with your hands.

4. Place three flat cooking bowls side by side, put flour in the first bowl, beaten eggs in the second bowl and in the third, semolina.

5. Pass the balls (gnudi) repeatedly through the flour, the eggs and semolina.

6. Fry the coated balls in a hot pan with white-fizzing butter. Roll the gnudi around in the pan until the butter colours brown.

7. Remove the pan from the heat.

8. Add the lemon peel, sea lavender and sage to the pan, but don't put the pan back on the heat.

9. After a few seconds it'll be ready to serve.

10. Steam the fish and season well with salt and pepper.

Smoked salmon sushi bowl

Preparation time

20 minutes

Ingredients

- Wasabi Mayonnaise

- 2 tbsp real mayonnaise

- 1 tbsp wasabi paste

- 1 tsp rice vinegar

Bowls

- 1 cup sushi rice cooked and cooled

- 2 sheets of nori (toasted seaweed) dampened

- 4 oz MSC certified smoked salmon

- 1 cup cucumber cut into matchsticks

- 1 avocado sliced

- 2 scallions sliced

- 1 tsp black sesame seeds

- soy sauce

Instructions

Wasabi Mayonnaise

1. In a small bowl, whisk together the mayonnaise, wasabi paste, and rice vinegar.

2. Refrigerate until ready to use.

Bowls

1. Divide rice between two bowls

2. With your fingers, dampen nori with water, and cut into strips.

3. Divide the nori between the two bowls.

4. Roll smoked salmon slices into cigar shapes and divide between the bowls

5. Top the bowls with avocado, cucumber slices and scallions.

6. Sprinkle each bowl with sesame seeds, and drizzle with wasabi mayonnaise

7. Serve with soy sauce on the side.

Tuna noodle caboodle

Preparation time

1 hour 30 minutes

Ingredients

- 1 tin of Scout Tuna in Olive Oil

- 1 pinch of salt

- 2 cups of elbow macaroni

- ¼ cups of salted butter

- ¼ cups of all purpose flour

- 2 tbsps of Old Bay seasoning

- 2 cups of whole milk

- 2 cups of mozzarella or provolone cheese

- ½ cup of frozen corn

- ½ cup of frozen peas

- ½ cup of frozen carrots

- 1 bag of a crunchy chip of your choice

Instructions

1. Preheat your oven to 350 degrees.

2. Bring a medium sized pot of water to a boil.

3. Add a pinch of salt and cook the macaroni noodles until they're very, very tender (15-20 minutes).

4. In another medium sized pot, melt your butter on low-medium heat and whisk in your flour.

5. When a nice almond colour begins to develop, add in your Old Bay seasoning and whole milk.

Whisk everything together and increase the heat to medium-high.

6. The sauce will begin to thicken.

7. Once your sauce has thickened, melt in all your cheese. Set aside.

8. Mix together your cheese sauce, noodles, corn, peas, carrots and Scout Tuna in Olive Oil into a oven-proof casserole dish.

9. Bake for 30 minutes, or until the top is bubbling and golden.

10. Remove your casserole from the oven, and crumble your chips on top.

11. Serve hot.

Lobster Polenta Bake

Preparation time

1 hour 15 minutes

Ingredients

- 4 Cups Chicken stock

- 1 cup 35% cream

- 2 Cups Polenta

- 1 tin of Scouts' Lobster

- 1 cup of Grated aged white cheddar

- 2 TBSP cold butter

- Salt to taste

- Lemon to garnish (optional)

Instructions

1. In a medium size pot, bring Chicken stock and 35% Cream to a simmer. Season to taste.

2. Slowly whisk in your Cornmeal or stone ground polenta slowly and gently until well blended and starting to become thick.

3. In an oven proof dish, pour the polenta into the dish, top with one tin of Scouts' Lobster and a generous topping of aged white cheddar

4. Bake at 350 degrees C for 35-45 minutes, or until bubbling and golden brown

5. Remove from oven and scoop a generous portion and garnish with some fresh cheddar and
a little lemon wedge

Tuna Salad with Couscous

Preparation time

20 minutes

Ingredients

- 4 oz can MSC certified tuna (broken into chunks)

- ¾ cup uncooked Moroccan couscous

- 1 cup vegetable broth

- ¼ tsp Kosher Salt

- 2 tsp grapeseed oil

- ½ red bell pepper (medium diced)

- 3 oz seeded red Kalamata olives

- 3 oz seeded green olives

- 2 tbsp Italian parsley (roughly chopped)

- 1 heirloom beefsteak tomato (medium diced)

- ½ hot house cucumber (medium diced)

- 3 preserved grape leaves (layer leaves, roll them tightly and "chiffonade"- cut into thin strips)

- Dressing Ingredients:

- ½ cup cider vinegar

- ¼ cup grapeseed oil

- 1 tbsp lemon juice

- 2 tbsp orange blossom honey

- Salt and pepper

Instructions

1. To make the couscous, add vegetable broth and grapeseed oil to a small saucepan; bring to a boil.

2. Stir in the couscous, cover, and remove from heat.

3. Let stand for five minutes, then fluff with fork, and set aside to cool.

4. To make the dressing, combine all dressing ingredients in a small glass bowl and incorporate thoroughly.

5. Season with salt and pepper to taste.

6. Plate by folding together the couscous, vegetables and desired amount of dressing in a large bowl and fluff.

7. Add the flakey chunks of tuna on top of a bed of couscous salad and drizzle remaining dressing over salad and tuna.

8. Garnish with fresh lime wedges, a sprinkle of parsley and fresh-cracked black pepper.

Fish red curry

Preparation time

40 minutes

Ingredients

- 170 grams fine egg noodles

- 1 tablespoon olive oil

- 1/3 cup peanut oil

- 500 grams MSC certified white fish such as hake or cod, cubed

- 2 garlic cloves, minced

- 6 spring onions, finely sliced

- 80 grams of Thai red curry paste

- 2 tablespoons soya sauce

- 1 tablespoon fish sauce

- 2 teaspoons chili flakes (or less if you don't like heat)

- Juice of 1 lime

- 2 tablespoons honey

- 400 ml of coconut milk

- 1 punnet sugar snaps

- 1 generous handle coriander

- 1 small pineapple, peeled and sliced into pieces

- 1/2 cup roasted peanuts

- Bean sprouts and lime for serving

Instructions

1. Cook the noodles in salted water as per packet instruction and set aside.

2. Add a glug of olive oil so your noodles don't stick when it comes time to serve.

3. Meanwhile, in a medium frying pan over medium heat add a drizzle of peanut oil.

4. Add the fish and sear on each side until just cooked through. Roughly 3-4 minutes.

5. If your pan isn't big enough do this in two batches.

6. Once ready remove from the pan and set aside on a plate.

7. In the same frying pan over medium heat add another dash of peanut oil. Add the spring onions and sauté for three minutes.

8. Add the curry paste and sauté for an additional two minutes releasing the flavours.

9. Add the soya sauce, fish sauce, chilli flakes, lime juice, honey, and cook for an additional two

minutes stirring often and releasing the fragrant flavours.

10. Add the coconut milk and stir in with the rest of the ingredients.

11. Allow the sauce to simmer for 5-10 minutes on reduced heat. This will allow the flavours to develop.

12. Once the sauce is ready add the sugar snaps and fish to the sauce.

13. Cook until the fish has warmed through and the sauce has thickened.

14. Roughly five to ten minutes.

15. Once ready remove from the heat and stir in the coriander.

16. To serve, add the noodles to your bowls and pour over the curry.

17. Top off with coriander, pineapple, and peanuts for that extra crunch.

Crumbed hake baguette

Preparation time

40 minutes

Ingredients

- 500g box of crumbed hake fillets

- 2 baguettes

- 1 head of fennel, thinly sliced

- 5-6 cornichons or cocktail gherkins, finely chopped

- 1 small red onion, thinly sliced

- 1 small head of iceberg lettuce, shredded

- Tangy mayonnaise

- Coarse ground sea salt and black pepper

- Lemon wedges, to serve

Instructions

1. Preheat the oven to 220°C and line a baking sheet with foil or baking paper.

2. Lightly drizzle each crumbed hake fillet with a little olive oil and arrange on the baking sheet.

3.   Arrange the sliced fennel around the fillets and drizzle with olive oil and salt and pepper.

4. Grill the hake and fennel for 20-25 minutes.

5.   Combine 50ml of mayonnaise with the chopped cocktail gherkins and season to taste.

6.   Slice each baguette in half lengthways, spreading the base of each baguette liberally with the gherkin mayonnaise and pile on the shredded lettuce.

7. Scatter over the sliced onion and top each baguette with the grilled fennel and hake fillets.

8. Close up the sandwiches with the other half of baguette and secure with cocktail skewers.

9. Serve the sandwiches with lemon wedges for squeezing over the fish.

Crispy Potato Cakes with Herb Marinated Cold Water Shrimp

Preparation time

1 hour

Ingredients

- 3 large russet potatoes

- 1 medium spanish or white onion

- 340 g (3/4 lb) MSC certified cold water shrimp, thawed and drained

- 200 g (3/4 cup) full-fat sour cream

- 1 small bunch each of fresh thyme, fresh basil, fresh flat-leaf parsley, fresh oregano

- 2 cloves of garlic

- ¼ cup of olive oil

- Zest and juice of 1 lemon

- Salt to taste

- Capers, caper berries, microgreens, or pickled onions (optional garnish suggestions)

Instructions

1. Make sure shrimp are thawed and drained. Remove any excess liquid and store in fridge until you're ready to use.

2. Peel onion. Using the rough side of a cheese grater, grate into a bowl.

3. Grate the washed but not peeled potatoes using the same side of the cheese grater.

4. Add to bowl with onions. Tip: grating the onion first helps keep the potatoes from oxidizing.

5. Season grated mixture with a little bit of salt and mix together well.

6. The mixture will start to weep liquid once you add salt – don't worry, that's exactly what you are looking for.

7. Preheat your frying pan to medium heat and get your baking sheet and spatula ready to go.

8. Using your hands, take a bit of the mixture, about the size of a ping pong ball, and squeeze as much liquid out of it as you can.

9. Place this in the heated frying pan and press down so it is flat.

10. Continue to do so until the pan is filled with potato cakes.

11. Cook until golden brown on both sides and add more oil if they start to stick to the pan.

12. Set aside cooked potato cakes and let rest while you prepare the cold water shrimp.

13. Roughly chop all the herbs, zest and squeeze juice from the lemon and mix together in a bowl.

14. Add the olive oil, cold water shrimp, and season to taste.

15. To assemble, place potato cakes on a platter, top generously with sour cream and add the final touch – a generous spoonful of the marinated shrimp.

16. Garnish and serve.

Haddock and broccoli bake

Preparation time

40 minutes

Ingredients

• 30ml (2 tablespoons) olive oil

- 2.5ml (½ teaspoon) smoked paprika

- Pinch of ground turmeric

- 30ml (2 tablespoons) wheat cake flour

- 625ml (2 ½ cups) warm low-fat milk

- 5ml (1 teaspoon) fish spice

- Flaked sea salt and fresh black pepper

- 60ml (¼ cup) grated parmesan cheese, optional

- 60ml (¼ cup) grated mozzarella cheese, plus 30 ml extra

- 60ml (¼ cup) grated mature cheddar cheese , plus 30 ml extra

- 500g (1 box) frozen MSC certified haddock, thawed and cut into chunks

- 400g long stem broccoli stems

- 5ml (1 teaspoon) freshly black pepper

Instructions

1. For the sauce: Preheat the oven to 180º C and in a large non-stick saucepan, heat the flora margarine until melted, add the spices and cook for 30 seconds.

2. Whisk in the flour little at a time to create a roux. Take the pan off the heat and whisk in the warm milk. Place back on the heat and continue whisking.

3. Bring to the boil and simmer for 8 minutes, still whisking. Season the with fish spice, salt and pepper and stir until well combined.

4. Switch off the stove and add the different cheeses, stir until melted. Pour the sauce in an oven proof baking dish.

5. Place the thawed and pat-dried haddock chunks on top of the sauce followed by broccoli stems, lightly season the broccoli with a pinch of salt. Sprinkle with the extra cheddar and mozzarella cheese.

6. Bake in the oven for 20 minutes until fish is cooked, until golden and bubbling. Serve with fresh dill and lime wedges and starch of your choice.

Creamy mussels with 'courgetti' pasta

Preparation time

27 minutes

Ingredients

- Courgette pasta

- 30ml (2 tablespoons) olive oil

- 2 cloves garlic, crushed

- 5ml (1 teaspoon) fresh thyme, chopped

- 8 large courgettes, sliced into long thin strips using a spiked vegetable peeler

- Pinch of flaked sea salt

- Creamy mussels

- 15ml (1 tablespoon) butter

- 2 cloves garlic, crushed

- 2.5ml (½ teaspoon) mustard powder

- 15ml (1 tablespoon) whole-grain mustard

- 125ml (½ cup) good-quality chicken stock

- 180ml (¾ cup) low-fat milk

- 30ml (2 tablespoons) crème fraîche

- 4 x 115 g tinned MSC certified mussels in oil

Serve with

- Toasted ciabatta slices

- Charred lime

Instructions

1. For the 'courgetti' pasta: heat the oil in a large saucepan and sauté the garlic for 1 minute, add the chives and thyme and cook for a further minute.

2. Add the 'courgetti' pasta and stir-fry for 2–3 minutes, until al dente, taking care not to overcook them. Remove from heat.

3. To make the creamy mussels: heat the butter until melted for 1 minute.

4. Add the mustard powder and whole-grain mustard and stir for about 30 seconds.

5. Whisk in the stock and milk and bring to the boil.

6. Simmer for 5 minutes.

7. Add the crème fraîche and stir until dissolved.

8. Add the canned mussels and cook for 2 minutes.

9. To serve: divide the pasta 'courgetti' into four soup bowls. Pour the creamy mussel sauce in the bowl and serve with toasted bread, a squeeze of lime and sprinkle with chili flakes.

Roasted mackerel and mixed tomatoes

Preparation time

22 minutes

Ingredients

- 2 fillets of MSC certified mackerel, cleaned

- Flaked sea salt and black pepper

- 250g fresh exotic cherry tomatoes, some halved and some sliced

- A handful of fresh basil leaves

- A handful of fresh dill

Spicy apricot and harissa glaze

- 60ml (1/4 cup) apricot jam

- 15ml (1 tablespoon) harissa paste

- 30ml (2 tablespoons) fish stock

- Juice of ½ lime

- 15ml (1 tablespoon) fresh dill, chopped

Instructions

1. Preheat the oven to 200°C and line a baking sheet with baking paper.

2. Pat-dry the mackerel with paper towel and place it skin-side down on the prepared baking tray.

3. Season with salt and pepper.

4. In a small saucepan over high heat, place all the glaze ingredients together, except for the dill and stir vigorously until combined.

5. Bring to the boil, reduce the heat to medium and simmer for 3 minutes.

6. Stir in the dill and turn off the heat.

7. Using a basting brush, generously smear the mackerel with the glaze.

8. Add the tomatoes.

9. Lightly season with sea salt and bake for 10 minutes until the fish is cooked.

10. Remove from the oven and garnish with fresh basil leaves and dill.

11. Enjoy it with mash or as a wrap or serve with salad.

Wild crispy skin salmon with white bean and coriander puree

Preparation time

1 hour 30 minutes

Ingredients

- 2 x 170g MSC certified Wild John West salmon fillets, skin left on but scaled, pin-boned

- 4 baby beetroot

- olive oil, for drizzling

- sea salt flakes and freshly

- ground black pepper

- 60 ml balsamic vinegar

- 2 x 400g tins cannellini beans, drained and rinsed

- 1 garlic clove

- juice of 1 lemon

- 120 ml vegetable stock

- 1/2 bunch of coriander, leaves and stems

- 1/4 bunch of dill, finely chopped

- 4 tablespoons Basic Mayonnaise

- 4 slices of sourdough bread, cut into 1.5cm cubes

- 1 handful of micro herbs

- 1 lemon, cut into wedges

Instructions

1. Preheat the oven to 180°C.

2. Place the beetroot in an ovenproof dish, dress with a little olive oil and season with salt and pepper.

3. Roast in the oven for 45 minutes, or until tender. Set aside to cool, then peel and cut into wedges.

4. Place the beetroot and balsamic vinegar in a bowl and set aside.

5. Place the cannellini beans in a food processor, add the garlic, half the lemon juice and a drizzle of olive oil and blitz to combine.

6. Loosen with the stock and whiz until nice and smooth.

7. Add the coriander and continue to blitz until smooth.

8. Transfer to a small saucepan and heat through.

9. Season to taste, and keep warm.

10. Combine the dill with the mayonnaise and season with salt, pepper and the remaining lemon juice.

11. To make the croutons, pan fry the sourdough cubes with a little olive oil and salt in a frying pan over medium heat until golden brown.

12. Drain on paper towel.

13. Rub the salmon flesh with a little olive oil and season the skin with salt. Leave for 10 minutes to draw the excess moisture out of the skin.

14. Pat the skin dry using kitchen towel and season again with salt.

15. Heat a heavy-based frying pan over a high heat, add the salmon, skin side down, and fry for 3 minutes.

16. Turn and cook for another 2 minutes.

17. To serve, arrange the salmon, puree, beetroot and croutons on the plate. Serve the dill mayonnaise in a bowl on the side.

18. Garnish with red micro herbs and a wedge of lemon.

Mediterranean Tuna and Cannelini Bean Salad

Preparation time

20 minutes

Ingredients

- 1 shallot

- 2 cloves garlic

- 220g tinned cannelini beans

- 300g MSC certified tinned tuna

- 1 tsp thyme leaves

- 1 small jar sun dried tomatoes

- 1/2 lemon

- 3 tbsp chopped basil

- 85ml extra virgin olive oil

Instructions

1. Gently sweat down the shallots and garlic in the olive oil, until soft and translucent.

2. Add the beans and, carefully as not to break them up too much, warm through.

3. Add the tuna, tomatoes and thyme. Continue to warm.

4. Finish with the fresh basil and lemon juice.

5. Serve alongside crusty bread or some fresh bitter leaves like rocket or watercress.

Asian salmon cakes

Preparation time

25 minutes

Ingredients

- 2 cans MSC certified Sockeye Salmon (213 gram cans)

- 2 tbsp soy sauce

- 2 garlic cloves, crushed and diced finely

- 1 tbsp ginger, peeled and grated

- 1/4 cup green onions, finely diced

- 2 tbsp lemon juice

- 2 large eggs

- 1/2 cup panko

- 1/4 cup sesame seeds

- vegetable oil for frying

Instructions

1. Open 2 cans of MSC certified salmon and drain all liquid

2. In a large bowl, combine salmon, soy sauce, garlic, ginger, and green onions and combine

3. Add lemon juice

4. Add 2 eggs and mix until combined

5. In a separate bowl, add panko and sesame seeds

6. In a large cast iron pan, add oil and heat to medium/low heat

7. Roll each fish cake and flatten to a small disc, coat with panko and sesame seed on both sides

8. Pan fry each fish cakes, about 2 minutes on each side or until golden brown

9. Serve with green onions, red chili peppers and garlic chili sauce as garnish if you like.

Cape Malay-style pickled hake

Preparation time

40 minutes

Ingredients

• MSC certified Deep-sea hake fillets, cut into portions

• 2 tbsp olive oil

• 5 large onions, cut into thin rings

• 1 x 3 cm piece fresh ginger, grated

- 4 cloves garlic, crushed

- 5 tspn mild curry powder

- 2 tspn tumeric

- 6 bay leaves

- 1 tspn whole allspice or allspice powder

- 1 tspn coriander seeds

- 1 tspn whole cumin or cumin powder

- 1 litre white vinegar

- 300 g sugar

- Sea salt and freshly ground black pepper

- Flour, for dusting

Instructions

1. In a stainless-steel saucepan over a medium heat, add 1 T oil and, when hot, gently sauté the onion until translucent.

2. Add the ginger, garlic and spices and fry gently for a few minutes, or until fragrant.

3. Add the vinegar and sugar and stir until the sugar has dissolved.

4. Simmer for 20 minutes.

5. Meanwhile, dust the fish with the seasoned flour and pat off any excess.

6. Heat 1 T oil in a heavy-based frying pan and, when hot, fry the fish until golden but still succulent.

7. Place a layer of fish in a deep sterile glass or non-metallic container and pour a little of the hot sauce over it, to cover.

8. Continue layering fish and sauce until all the fish is covered.

9. Cool, then chill until ready to serve.